How Will I Get Rid Of My Hernia?
Without Surgery!

Detailed Instructions

Carsten Bachmeyer

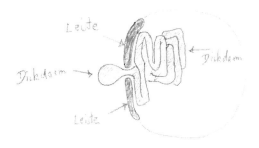

How Will I Get Rid Of My Hernia?
Without Surgery!

Detailed Instructions

Carsten Bachmeyer
E-Mail: leistenbruch-selber-heilen@gmx.de

Copyright © 2012 Author: Carsten Bachmeyer. All rights reserved.
Produced and Published by:
Books on Demand GmbH, Norderstedt
ISBN 978-3-8448-0400-3

Cover Photo by Piotr Marcinski,
Fotolia

The use of the book and the realization of the information given are undertaken expressly at the reader's own risk. Liability claims against the publishing company and the author for material, health and immaterial damages, caused by the use or non-use of information respectively the use of faulty and/or incomplete information are strictly excluded. Consequently legal rights and compensation claims are excluded. This book including all contents was elaborated with utmost care. The publishing company and the author, however, do not assume any responsibility for the topicality, correctness, completeness and quality of the provided information. Misprints and errors cannot be completely excluded. The publishing company and the author assume liability neither for the topicality, correctness and completeness of the book's contents nor for printing mistakes. Neither legal responsibility nor any liability for incorrect data and their consequences will be taken by the publishing company respectively the author.

This book including all its components is protected by copyright. Any utilisation outside the tight limits of the Copyright Act is not allowed and punishable without the prior consent of the publishing company. This especially refers to copying, translations, microfilming and saving and processing in electronic systems.

For Mia...
and all other people who want to get rid of their
hernia without surgery.

„Be courageous and make use of your own mind."

Immanuel Kant

„The phenotype of a human individual is a 100% reflection of his genotype."

Carsten Bachmeyer

Contents

11 Foreword

13 The Mystery of Non-Healing Hernia

16 Introduction

24 Hernia – A Profitable Business

27 3 Illustrations of Hernia

30 The Long Way to Knowledge

37 Theories Referring to Evolutionary Biology

39 Attitudes of a Family Doctor

41 Detailed Instructions for Treating Hernia (without surgery)

43 Instruction for Reducing resp. Removing the Pressure on the Groin

46 Three Days-Examples of Daily Nutrition

52 For Vegetarians

53 Putting on the Truss

56 Instructions of Putting on the Truss

68 Groin Pad

69 Short Summary

71 Important Things to be Considered by All Means In Your Everyday Life

73 Hernia on Both Sides

77 Further Examples of Meals

86 The Advantage of Hernia: It Is Visible!

Foreword

A detailed instruction for the treatment of your hernia is given in this book. Hernia need not be operated! Comparable to a torn ligament or a flesh wound it will heal by itself, if the groin is brought back in its usual position. This is achieved by a dietary change and the use of the special truss.

Thanks to the dietary change the intestine will no longer prevent the healing process of the groin.

Your groin will have healed and strengthened after you have followed the diet plan and used the special truss for a few months. Unless it was tried to doctor with your hernia according to the traditional medicine, you will be one of the lucky persons who will recover quickly. But also patients whose hernia was repaired by use of a mesh or whose mesh had to be removed again (and there will certainly be quite a lot of such patients) and those who are suffering from a relapse (operated hernia ruptured again) need not be worried. On the contrary they should be herewith inspired to think about the ideas given in this book. It's not too late (mostly)!

References to the evolutionary biology and nutrition science only serve as general considerations and information. The opinions of recognized experts - particularly in the nutrition science - differ substantially. It will probably take some decades to discover the "truth".

But it is known for certain that adhering to the diet plan of this book during the hernia treatment will lead to a healed groin (if the truss is worn in addition to the diet plan) …. this result will be achieved within a few weeks resp. months.

The instructions for treating hernia are the main topic of this book. It works! Give it a chance! It should be worth a trial.

The risk of an intestinal incarceration in the groin is decreased after a few days!

You've got the chance – it's up to you now!

In the introduction I will describe the aberrations and experiences which helped me getting the idea of this way of hernia treatment. This is contradictory to the opinion of all so-called experts who all unanimously maintained that it would be impossible to heal hernia without surgery.

The Mystery of Non-Healing Hernia

Why does hernia come into being? Why doesn't it heal by itself?

The groin cannot heal for the following reason: Comparable to piercing, the large intestine daily pushes itself from the abdomen to the outside by passing the ruptured groin. After a piercing is removed from the puncture, the tissue will close again at this body site. If the piercing is, however, left in the tissue, it can of course not close. This is also applicable to groin and intestine, with the intestine playing the role of the piercing. Consequently the intestine must be prevented from penetrating the groin every day, so that the groin can close in its usual anatomic position. But how shall this work without the use of complicated surgical instruments? The reply will be given later.

In our case the intestine is the groin's major enemy. Being penetrated by the intestine every day, the groin is given no chance of healing.

During the digestion of a single meal in which food was mixed (that means carbohydrates and proteins) up to 18 litres of gas are produced in the intestine.

18 litres of gas are quite a lot. The intestine is extremely bloated and the physical forces impacting the groin are enormous. Thus the groin is exposed to a great load every day and will sooner or later give way to it.... at least in case of every third or forth human being on earth.

I maintain that the intestines of human beings in all civilized industrial states of the world have lost their natural size and have substantially exceeded by bloating. Due to its unnatural increased volume (mainly caused by denatured carbohydrates), the bloated intestine will continuously press from the inside on the groin. If the intestine was, however, reduced to its natural volume, it would no longer penetrate the ruptured groin which in turn could close.

Thanks to the diet plan listed in this book the intestine's volume will be reduced substantially. If the diet plan is followed, the hernia sac will become smaller day by day. You will state this immediately in the course of the first days. The hernia sac may be compared with an "intestine-meter" showing the de-/increasing volume of the intestine.

Due to the dietary change your groin is given the opportunity to heal and to form firm tissue, as the intestine no longer penetrates it daily. The intestine has meanwhile returned to its original volume (without producing harmful gases) and does not prevent any more the groin during its healing.

That's the big mystery of the non-healing groin.

If additionally a slight external pressure – generated by the particular truss - is applied to the hernia, you will soon get rid of your hernia problem.

Introduction

In 1999 I contracted hernia on both sides. Due to a bad gastrointestinal virus I was violently ill. As I had to vomit several times, enormous pressure was put on the groin. As a consequence both groins ruptured during that night. The hernia on the right-hand side (approx. plum-sized) healed by itself after approx. 6 weeks, while the hernia on the left side continuously increased. Finally it featured a lemon-sized buckling which remained constant for more than 10 years. At that time the doctors recommended an immediate operation pointing out the risk of a possible intestinal incarceration and its life-threatening complications. But an operation was out of a question for various reasons.

First of all I did not know which operation method would be the best; secondly I refused a mesh as I did not agree having a foreign matter in my body for the rest of my life. In my opinion a foreign matter which will cause problems and probably will have to be removed by surgery (there are hospitals which are specialised on the removal of meshes) was certainly no alternative. I even considered the mesh as proof of the incompetent traditional medicine. 5% - 10% anguished victims have been recorded – that's not a high success rate. If you knew that 5% - 10% of all planes would crash, would you still go by plane? I wouldn't!

When I lied down at night, the hernia sac disappeared. Having got up in the morning, a large, firm hernia sac immediately showed up again.

Everything was going fine for 10 years..... until the groin ruptured further and the size of the hernia sac enlarged drastically. The hernia sac was as large as an avocado or a medium-sized apple. At this time - at the very latest - I was forced to act. I wondered: Will the hernia increase even further, ranging from the scrotum to the neck? When will the groin on the other side rupture? It seemed to be only a matter of time, until my whole body would suffer from the weak connective tissue. The next day I right away went to see my family doctor who – as expected – recommended an immediate operation. I saw two specialists in Berlin and Munich who both advised the immediate surgery as well.

I went to see numerous hospitals specialised in naturopathy and homeopaths. I was surprised that they all recommended an immediate operation. I researched in internet, met a lot of doctors and specialists, visited clinics and hospitals specialised in naturopathy. There was evidently no possibility to avoid surgery due to lack of alternatives. I was prepared to take radical measures without knowing which measures would be appropriate.

I read books about eaters of raw food, miracle healers, traditional doctors, Atkin (meat diet), Wearland (bread diet) and thought of possible solutions to this problem.

I tried to get information about the food of human beings in natural and unspoiled surroundings, intending to adapt my food accordingly. But how should I get to know this in an entirely industrialised world?

The human being moved out of nature, having to pay now a great deal in consideration of the numerous invalids.

Each of the unlimited number of specialists, doctors and academics in nutrition science has an opinion – mostly a different than the others: 1000 specialists = 1000 different opinions. How should I form my own opinion in consideration of these substantially differing views? It was impossible to do so. I looked for a species whose genotype and phenotype are most similar to those of human beings and that lives in the wild without depending on human beings.

At this time I still thought having weak connective tissue which could be strengthened by perfect food, so that consequently my hernia would heal by itself. Later I realized that the hernia was not at all due to weak connective tissue, but to a quite different fact..... I will refer to it later.

I tried to find out the really typical food of a human being. What would he eat in wild natural surroundings, if he only followed his own instincts.... without being influenced by television advertising or dubious experts.

Considering all different and confusing statements of the experts, I was sure about one fact: Any creature that deviates from its typal food will fall ill sooner or later, which I remembered having been taught at school in the advanced class of biology and which I could understand according to observations and thoughts of my own. For example: a dolphin being exclusively fed with bread will fall ill very soon and die. A shark living only on alga would also sicken within short and turn to be non-viable. That's exactly the same in case of a lion being fed only with apples or a giraffe only living on meat.... they would all fall ill. Each species features its own typal food. If the creature deviates from this food, it will sicken and die.

To me, it therefore made a lot of sense to get an idea of the humans' typal food. Many people will now recommend asking a nutrition expert, biologist or doctor. And there's exactly a snag. If a believed in the experts' statements, I would probably now have an operation scar, possibly including shrunk testicles, and additionally would have never healed my hernia by myself.

It remains to be seen whether these considerations regarding dietetics are reasonable. But in case of treating the hernia they have been successful

I could only think of the chimpanzee with all its natural instincts and behaviour as example of a creature in the wild. With regard to phenotype and genotype there is no other creature on earth which is more similar to a human being.

Before I now continued to think intensely about dietary strategies, I was prepared to run an individual test by adopting the chimpanzee's food without any changes. I was up to execute my own medial experiment, regardless of any possible consequences for myself....

In the wild and natural surroundings the chimpanzee's consists of approx. 60% raw vegetables and fruit and 40% raw meat. For hygienic reasons I would of course not eat the meat raw.

In my view my connective tissue could be gradually strengthened by this type of food. I would have never expected the success to follow within days.... or even hours!

The progress in recovery had nothing to do with weak convective tissue. Maybe I did not suffer from weak convective tissue at all?

Applying my new „chimpanzee-diet" the avocado-sized hernia sac reduced to grape-size within 2 days. Furthermore it became very soft, after it had been really tight and firm before. Having in mind the numerous consultations of the last years, it seemed like a miracle that hernia could be healed so quickly WITHOUT SURGERY or that at least the risk of an intestinal incarceration could be eliminated.

I was very surprised of the dramatic and quick changing as consequence of the dietary change! As the hernia sac was so small and soft, it could be ligated. For reasons of "first aid" I instinctively took my winter scarf out of the wardrobe and put it around my hip. This worked very well, but I was still looking for a more optimal solution.

After my 10 years' hernia I had at least managed to bring the groin back into its original, anatomically correct position!!!

I bought some expensive trusses in an orthopaedic shop. They were extremely uncomfortable, giving pain and leaving unpleasant pressure marks on the skin. Some trusses even constricted the blood supply, while others featured a golf ball-sized knob which put painful pressure on the groin. Furthermore these trusses got out of place very easily and thus did not guarantee a stabilization of the hernia. The leather – most of the trusses are made of – is non-elastic and does not nestle to the body.

Therefore I again had to find a solution by myself. I again used by winter scarf and tried some different techniques. Since the beginning the scarf had always been a better solution than any of the expensive trusses bought in the orthopaedic shop. Finally I had found a technique of tying the scarf in such a way that the hernia opening was perfectly ligated.

At the latest at this time I knew that I would be able to heal my hernia by myself. I do not know why, but everything appeared to be logical. When I euphorically informed my family and friends accordingly, they all waved aside, smirking at me: "Everybody knows that hernia will never heal by itself ... Have an operation and that's it!" I was going against the tide, being disapproved by everybody.... but I continued pursuing my plan. Since I had changed my dietary, the hernia sac had disappeared ....and never appeared again.

I very strictly adhered to my own dietary instructions (chimpanzee-diet) and have always worn the scarf-belt except during sleeping. I do not know when my hernia had completely healed, but I think that the worst was over after 4-6 weeks. To be on the safe side I continued wearing the scarf-belt for another 3 months (approx.) (totally about 4 months). You get quickly used to the belt which you can put on/off without a few seconds.

Furthermore I was afraid of renouncing the belt and going outside without it. I was too frightened of the hernia re-appearing. I think that the groin had well closed already after 6-8 weeks... but in my view the special truss should be worn for a longer period, at least for 3 months. In contrast to the conventional trusses, which may have very bad side effects, you can wear the scarf-belt without any physical constraints. Therefore it makes no sense at all to stop wearing the scarf-belt too early.

But somehow you will have to leave the belt out. When I went outside for the first time without scarf-belt after approx. 4 months, it was a strange feeling. After having suffered from large hernia sac for 10 years, you can hardly believe of its sudden disappearance.

My hernia healed within a very short time. Since 2009 I have been fully fit and relieved from the hernia .... despite physical load. I do power training with heavy weights, go jogging regularly, eat the usual home cooking and I am perfectly healthy. I myself have healed the 10 years old, avocado-sized hernia without surgery.

Hernia – A Profitable Business

Every year approx. 250.000 people in Germany contract hernia. Converting this to Euro leads to a very profitable business for the pharmaceutical industry and the participating doctors. Unless this surgery was required, the finances of the pharmaceutical industry would be at a low ebb of billions. Consequently the doctors unambiguously recommend an operation!

You are completely helpless in the face of the traditional medicine including its „surgery-enthusiastic" doctors. There is nothing more beautiful to them than surgery. They have learnt how to do it.... they want to make use of it. You are almost urged to an operation, especially by calling your attention to the risk of a life-threatening intestinal incarceration. Panic-stricken, you have hardly time to think and only wish to go through the operation as soon as possible. Please be advised that in most cases the risk of an intestinal incarceration will decrease within 2-5 days after the dietary change. It can be so easy!

The following questions now arise: How reasonable is such an operation and which implant (mesh) will be the best? How long will it take until I will contract hernia on the other side? Can it be assured that the repaired hernia will not break up again? Who will ensure you of not suffering from pain after surgery? Nothing to say of its dramatic side effects such as shrunken testicles or even loss of testicles in addition to the implications of anaesthesia and surgery-shock from which your body will suffer. The number of harmed operated persons must be immense. There are thousands of reports about this topic, among others in the „Spiegel". If you really believe that it is a harmless and banal routine operation, you must have become a victim of the traditional medicine's propaganda. A hernia operation is not easy at all and rather risky. Beside the necessity of exposing the spermatic cord, important nerve tracts are located directly at the surgical cut.

The keyhole surgery (nowadays many „experts" are crazy about it – especially the media are very fond of the minimal-invasive method which is supposed to be innovative) is the most dangerous of all operation methods. Only few people know that the most serious complications appear during this type of surgery, which is moreover extremely stressful for the organism.

Real experts only apply the keyhole method in exceptional cases due to the proportionally enormous risks.

Now let's deal with the real topic of this book, i.e. the following question:
CAN HERNIA HEAL BY ITSELF? By itself? Not really..... as you need to assist the healing ...at least for approx. 2 – 4 months. You have to pursue your aim consistently and resolutely.

Neither in the internet nor by your doctor, will you be given a positive reply whether hernia can be healed without surgery. The pharmaceutical industry determines the topics a prospective doctor will be taught at university by mainly pursuing financial purposes. Unfortunately the well-being of the patients is only very occasionally the most important aspect. It is imperative to follow and achieve a tightly calculated economic efficiency.

Basically, the doctor is nothing but a marionette of pharmaceutical industry – a graduated fellow-runner.

I really trash doctors with these statements, but I have no other clue why the simplest medical facts are complicated and why suffering and pain are often favoured instead of removed. I expect a doctor from helping me instead of intensifying my discomfort, no matter how much money he will make out of my treatment. After all, he has taken the Hippocratic Oath!

Furthermore I had expected a doctor from offering alternatives for surgery, as i.e. the therapy which is described in this book. How can it happen that I am able to develop such a therapy in contrast to innumerable first-class medical experts all over the world?

Medical science is a business. Healing hernia without operation means that no money can be earned!

3 Illustrations of Hernia

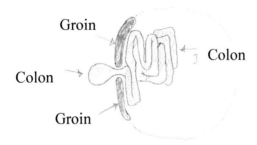

That's how hernia looks like. The hernia sac is formed mostly by the colon or small intestine. It repeatedly penetrates the groin, thus preventing a natural closing of the hernia gap.

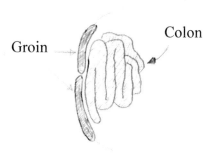

That's how it looks like when you go sleeping and lie on your back. The hernia sac disappears and the intestine moves back into the abdomen. The groin is back to its natural anatomy (without being closed).

If you lied on your back for 2-4months without getting up once, your groin would heal by itself. But it is not recommendable to do so.

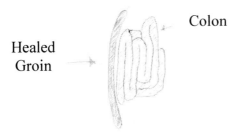

That's how your groin will look after approx. 2-6 months under the precondition that you have followed the instructions of this book.

The groin has closed again being as stable and firm as before.

The Long Way to Knowledge

Of course you may ask how I have got the idea of this method of treatment. Am I really the only person on earth who has found a way of healing hernia without surgery? It seems so according to internet research and discussions with doctors. Ask any doctor..... with a certainty of 100% you will be told that hernia will NEVER heal by itself.

Searching the truth is extremely difficult.... almost impossible. Nevertheless I am of the opinion that it is worthwhile to follow this laborious way to challenge things instead of simply believing what is said to be true. In former times the earth was believed to be flat. But this was not true although it had been maintained and believed by everybody. I do not consider the truth as a further way of faith as for example traditional medicine, Buddhism, Koran, Christianity, Islam and so on, but far more as a natural constant, such as for example: light velocity, number pi, round earth theory (not flat), theorem of Pythagoras or 1 + 1 = 2, infinity of universe and so on.

If you are disapproved by all doctors on earth and all fellow human beings, while being convinced of their being wrong, you need a lot of energy to starting re-testing things and to find new, unexplored approaches. Maybe a combination of events in my life initiated me in finding a way of healing hernia without surgery.
Since I was 30 years old, I suffered from a painful prostatitis. Due to this illness I could no longer take part in the usual social life. At night I had to get to the toilet up

to 15 times. I could no longer sleep and always had the feeling of a having a golf ball in my colon. I suffered at every step I took, but no doctor was able to help me. During seven years I went to see more than twenty urologists – at the end only experts. But even these specialists in urology (traditional medicine) were not able to prescribe the correct antibiotics. I was given antibiotics which did not even penetrate the prostate tissue. At that time my prostate was seized with bacteria of the type Enterococcus Faecalis. But the prescribed antibiotics did not work on the Gram-positive bacteria of the type Enterococcus Faecalis.

Being left entirely alone with my illness, I was on the verge of having removed the prostate in an operation. After extensive researches I, however, quickly gave up this intention. After approx. 5 years I managed to trace – assisted by the university hospital in Gießen – the antibiotic which was suitable for me: Levofloxacin. I went to my family doctor to have this medicament prescribed. About 3 days later my 6 years' prostatitis had dissolved into nothing. I was completely free of pain. It was almost a miracle and for about 24 hours I was the luckiest person on earth. During the antibiotic therapy the bacteria unfortunately returned (on 5th day) so that I again suffered from my prostatitis. The bacterium Enterococcus Faecalis had chronically seized my prostate.

The bacteria set up a so-called biofilm so that they could protect themselves against the antibiotics. If this medicament had been prescribed in the early phase of my illness..... in the acute stage....I could have saved me all trouble and stress. But the first medical specialist, I went to see, prescribed codlins-and-cream tea which helped me to get bad stomach aches.

After an odyssey of 6 years I accidentally met a doctor of a private clinic in Berlin. Compared with all other doctors, his statement most impressed me. According to him there was not much that could be done and I most probably would have to suffer from it lifelong. Like numerous patients I would have to take antibiotics every day. At the latest in this moment I realized that I had to find a new way. At least this doctor was honest and refrained from doctoring with me (i.e. cystoscopy, PSA-value, uro-flow-machine, punching out prostate tissue for laboratory tests and so on).

I spent all my energy to find solutions for my problem. I read all specialist literature pertaining to this topic. As a dog biting in its own tail, the traditional medicine could not help me at all. I tried to heal my body with food and sport (as it is nowadays usual in cancer therapies): endurance run every day and a great number of products from pharmacists (spending approx. 400 Euro per month for them), such as for example vitamin E, vitamin C, micronutrients and dietary supplements. I somewhat followed the theories of Prof. Strunz, the so-called „runner pope". While I was jogging, my prostate hurt me with every step.

It was a catastrophe and did not improve. After 3 months of "pharmacies' therapy" I by chance read in Prof. Strunz's book about a 119 years old doctor who had always been fit and never fell until the end of his life. This made me very curios. This old doctor was none other than Dr. Norman W. Walker. I now tried to get to know all details about this man and to buy all of his books. It was very difficult to buy this literature in Germany, but I eventually got them. I read the first of his books in a single night.

Everything that I had always known was written there black on white. Put down by a man who had never fallen ill, who still had had all his teeth and who peacefully died at the age of 119 years without pain, without tubes and above all without traditional medicine. He fed himself exclusively on raw food. The same night I went into my kitchen to throw away everything: spaghetti, bread, sugar, rice, instant meals, frozen meat, sausage salad with salad cream, jam, hazelnut spread ..... all this food was thrown into the waste bin.

From now on (year 1998) I was prepared to take consequential steps. Finally!!!! I again had a specific goal in mind that was worth being followed. From now on, I spent about 1200 DM/ 600 EUR per month for buying raw food in a health-food shop. Every day I squeezed approx. 1,5 l orange juice and approx. 4 l carrot juice..... sometimes even 6 l. I fed myself exclusively on raw food. After about 3 weeks I needn't go to the toilet at night and could sleep through! I had never thought that food would have such a striking influence on body respectively health. I turned to be a "raw food preacher"; I managed to take part in social life and was entirely healthy again. Today I have to point out that I am not convinced of feeding oneself 100% on raw food, although nutrition and food play a very important role in the hernia treatment.

It is important to inform you about all these details so that you can understand how I have got the idea of a hernia therapy without surgery. Without having suffered from the prostatitis, I would not have had this important knowledge and would have undergone a hernia operation. But thanks to this previous knowledge, I could look for and find an alternative solution.

I have been living with my lemon-sized hernia without any problems for eight years.

During this time I could do all kinds of sport with 100% load. I still went jogging, did power training and heavy physical gardening. The hernia got sometimes worse..... sometimes better. After having eaten for example much bread with cheese, the hernia hardened and caused pain. It was so painful that I had to lie down on my back until the hernia had disappeared in my abdomen. Eating unbalanced and one-sided (for example only fruits), the ailments didn't trouble me too much. But it was the same every morning: After I had got up, the hernia sac reappeared and became visible after it had penetrated the groin. You can certainly well imagine that the hernia sac was disturbing in numerous circumstances. It also continuously led to irregular bowel movements. This, however, would not have bothered me a lot.

In November 2009 the groin further ruptured. The uncomfortable feeling in the groins intensified. In this moment I realized that the size of a hernia was no constant. I had always thought until that time that due to anatomic circumstances the groin could not further rupture. I had been wrong. On the internet I saw hernias being as large as a baby. I assumed that my raw vegetables diet could not do anything about my hernia and that I had to accept the fact to have a surgery. Consequently I looked for various operation methods as for example keyhole surgery (minimal-invasive), operation according to Shouldice and of course thousands of various mesh operations including their advantages and disadvantages. Shortly after I was sure that a mesh would not be an alternative at all.
No long-term studies about these meshes are available. Specialists of large and famous clinics are very sceptical about these operations in which meshes are implanted. The side effects of all surgery variations did not seem to be a really good alternative. A very high number of cases in which patients suffer from substantial complications remain undetected.

Furthermore I think it is a very bad feeling if you are degraded by doctors to be mentally ill in consideration of your silicone testis, lots of pain and a continuously reappearing hernia. This is the typical behaviour of doctors who do not know how to continue.

I read about experimental projects/results of various clinics in which the groin was thoroughly examined. As for example: the groin can resist the six-fold pressure which strong cough puts on it (but these examinations were carried out with dead tissue, that means with dead bodies); the female connective tissue in the groin region is six times stronger than that of men. A ruptured groin looks like an old cleaning cloth which is continuously fraying in its middle so that the hole is getting larger and larger. Although I read a lot about it, I could not find exactly what I was looking for.

But finally I found a very interesting statement which could have also come to my mind. On his internet page a professor commented about hernia as follows: „If it could be prevented that the intestine continuously penetrates the groin, the problem and fear of hernia would be solved for long".

In other words: If the intestine could be prevented from continuously penetrating the groin, the groin would be given the chance to heal. According to Chinese medicine a buckling body is a sign of excessive wrong food. This might be phrased a bit clumsy, but in my opinion it indirectly hits the nail on its head.

I personally cannot imagine that nature – due to its incompetence – will allow every third or forth human being on earth to burst.

Removing hernia by surgery would not remove its real and actual cause. This means: If the cause is not tackled, further problems will occur – it's only a matter of time. I considered hernia as a sign of having done something basically wrong, according to my own theory.......

Theories Referring to Evolutionary Biology

The evolutionary biology deals – among others – with the terms „phenotype" and "genotype" of creatures. While „phenotype" refers to the outward appearance of creatures, „genotype" describes the genetics (DNA).

In the field of bionics engineers try to pick up a great deal of reasonable facts from nature and to transform them into techniques. Particularly the bionics pays utmost attention to the phenotype.

Think about the following simple example: Comparing a racing car (i.e. a Lamborghini) with a tractor, you can recognize from the phenotype that the Lamborghini can drive fast, while the tractor is rather slow. Thus it is able to find out the vehicles' performance on basis of their phenotypes. If this statement is applied to animals, you can well imagine the giraffe eating the leaves (among others) of a tree in a height of 15 m. Looking, however, at a lion's teeth and mouth, you might conclude from the phenotype that the lion is a carnivore. A cow on the meadow is obviously no carnivore as it is too inactive and slow for catching mammals. Thus you can think about the typal food of a special creature on basis of its phenotype.

In the wild the chimpanzee only eats raw food like all other creatures in natural surroundings. Its food consists of 60% vegetables and fruit and 40% natural protein (i.e. ants, small mammals and so on). Apart from the dangers in the wild the chimpanzee is quite healthy with this kind of food. If this chimpanzee were taken to our civilisation and fed with our food (denatured, treated, dead food) such as bread, potatoes, sugar and so on, it would certainly suffer from the same illnesses like human beings: diabetes (10 millions of diabetics in Germany), osteoporosis (10 millions), caries, cancer, cardiovascular diseases and so on.

I maintain that the typal food can be well concluded from the chimpanzee's phenotype. As the human being's phenotype is very similar to that of the chimpanzee, I even daresay the typal food of chimpanzees and human beings is the same.

According to Mahatma Gandhi: "You shouldn't eat anything that can't be eaten raw."

Attitudes of a Family Doctor

According to my family doctor (and the general traditional medicine) the appendix in my body is entirely useless. It was, however, created by nature in millions of years during the evolution. But my family doctor who obviously suffers from extremely high blood pressure (I would have liked to help him with his problem) outshines nature (for some readers: he outshines God). Well... he is the doctor! He went to university! I thought „There is something wrong in our system" and did not say anything. He was not very interested in the fact that I myself healed my hernia. He just snidely waved aside, saying: „Well... may be." But before, he had stated that hernia would NEVER heal by itself and that it would be a life-threatening risk due to the danger of intestinal incarceration. That's the way my doctor presents himself to me.

During an experiment in Germany thousands of doctors were tested. A reporter pretended to be a patient with a fractured rib. One should think of a quick and clear diagnosis in this easy case, but only a single doctor out of 10 was able to make a correct diagnosis. By the way, doctors neither get older than their patients nor are they healthier. But nevertheless we are passively in their pocket, doing nearly everything we are told by them.

The intelligent practice of doctors is nowadays reflected by the numerous clinics which have specialised in removing the meshes. Removing a mesh is a far more complicated operation than implanting it. That's, however, somewhat smart as there is the chance of making double and triple money out of the anguished patients. This fact will continue to happen unless it is refused to be accepted. During the last years/decades there were an increasing number of hernia patients who faced great problems and suffered pain caused by these implants. In the past it was said that no long-term studies were available. Today it should be recommended to refrain from these meshes. I myself would never undergo a hernia operation and hope that you will take the same decision after having read this book.

Detailed Instructions for Treating Hernia (without operation)

In case of hernia the biggest problem is the colon's respectively thin intestine's permanent pressure on the groin. That means: the groin is continuously exposed to an abnormal load, having nothing to do with a weak connective tissue. If this internal pressure could be removed, the secret of hernia would be revealed.

This means: First of all you have to remove the abnormal pressure in your abdomen. If you are already suffering from hernia, the intestine will continue penetrating the groin so that it is never given the chance to heal. Even if you wore my special truss, no healing would be expected.

Thanks to the diet described in this book your intestine will diminish to its original, natural volume. Harmful gases will no longer be produced; furthermore flatulence - bloating the intestine and putting an enormous internal pressure on the groin - is avoided. The groin will no longer be penetrated by the unnaturally bloated intestine. This is the most important aspect of this kind of hernia treatment.

This means:

1. Remove the abnormal pressure in the abdomen (by dietary change)

2. Use the special truss after 3-4 days upon removal of the abnormal pressure

3. Follow the nutrition instructions for at least 2-6 months and wear the truss

    (The times are to be complied with variably ... the longer.... the better ... particular with reference to the diet).

Detailed Instructions for Reducing respectively Removing the Pressure on the Groin

You have to change your diet for approx. 2 – 4 months (even better 6 months). This book is not intended to be a nutrition guide. But if you want your hernia to heal by itself, you must have to adhere to the following dietary plan. It is forbidden to use any "inorganic" carbohydrate (denatured, processed carbohydrate). This means: no potatoes, no rice, no spaghetti or noodles, no oat flakes, no corn flakes, no bread, no nuts, no cereals, no legumes...
Furthermore you are not allowed to have any milk products, such as for example latte macchiato (alternatively better have some filtered coffee or coffee cream with very little condensed milk), no yoghurt, no cheese (unless in addition to salad; in that case you may only have very little cheese), no chocolate, no sauces, no chips......

Beer drinkers should know that beer is one of the drinks, bringing to you a high calorie and carbohydrate. Unless you succeed in substantially reducing your beer consumption, you take the risk that the intestine will remain bloated and that the hernia will not heal. Apart from that the same rules being valid for all other drinks are applicable: you should drink before the meals. After the meals you should wait for at least 2 – 3 hours before you drink plenty of liquids.

Second important point: Do not mix any food. This means: you are not allowed to have salad and meat at the same time, instead of that only salad or only meat. 4-6 hours should go by between the meals.

You are allowed to exclusively eat and drink the following food, but without mixing them: .

Meat, fresh fruit, fresh vegetables, eggs, coffee (without sugar), tea (without sugar), water, freshly squeezed fruit- and vegetable juices (never buy fruit juices in a supermarket as they are all pasteurized and processed). You are ONLY allowed to drink juices ON AN EMPTY STOMACH.... NEVER after a meal!!! Wait for at least 2-3 hours after a meat meal and 2 hours after a salad!

YOU ARE NOT ALLOWED TO MIX ANY FOOD!!!

Why shouldn't you to drink (resp. drink only little) after a meal?

Water and juice have passed the stomach within a few minutes, while meat rests in the stomach for a longer time, being slowly stomached. If you drank directly after a meal, the stomaching would be extremely prolonged and the pancreas would produce more digestive juices. Consequently gas production in the intestine would be intensified so that in turn the intestine would more frequently penetrate the groin, impacting the healing process.

Furthermore you are not allowed to drink too much and too quickly. If you quickly drank one litre in one go, a very high pressure would be put on your groin within a few minutes, which would substantially endanger the healing process.

Three Examples of Daily Nutrition

Day 1

In the morning:

    2   coffees (with little condensed milk)
    2   bananas
    2   dried figs

At lunch time:

    1   big fresh salad with
    2   tomatoes
    ½   cucumber
    1   avocado
    ½   pepper
          olive oil
    50g feta cheese (you are allowed to mix the same type of food as i.e. vegetables; in this case: cucumber, tomatoes and avocado).

In the evening:

approx. 250g – 450g meat (depending on your stature), the less the better (at least during these 3-6 months) with little herb butter or olive oil. BY NO MEANS may you eat side dishes. Only the pure meat without any salad and of course without any denatured carbohydrates (bread, rice, noodles....).

Day 2   (a day for vegetarians)

In the morning:

1	orange juice (freshly squeezed)
1	coffee (without sugar, little condensed milk or even better without milk)
2	grated carrots
1	squeezed banana
10	raisins
3	dried figs

At lunchtime:

1	freshly squeezed orange juice
1	big fruit salad

In the evening:

1	big Greek farmer salad with max. 60 g feta cheese (see above)
1 – 2	grated carrots with olive oil and little salt as dessert (30 min. after supper)

Day 3

In the morning:

    2   teas   (drink slowly, no large gulps)
    2-3   eggs with bacon

At lunchtime:

First drink, then eat (15-20 min. later):

    250 – 450 g   meat (without side dishes)

                              only with little herb butter and/or olive oil. After the meal, only drink very little ….. it's better to wait for 2-3 hours.

In the evening:

First drink a bit (for example water or some freshly squeezed juice, but not more ¼ - ½ l), eat 15-20 min. later

    200 - 450 g   meat or fish WITHOUT side dishes, only little herb butter (for example 50 g) or olive oil.
You will have 3 principal meals each day (in the morning, at lunch time, in the evening).

There should be at least 5 hours each between the meals. If you feel hungry during these 5 hours, you should stand firm, think of your groin and stay the course (keep in mind: it's only a limited time, hang on). If you are not at all able to stand firm, eat 2-3 dried fruits, not more (for example: 3 Medjool dates or 2-3 dried figs or bananas).

Some of you will have to change their life radically. But keep in mind that you have to stand firm only for a limited time. But if you return to your previous dietary habits afterwards, the groin will be exposed to increased pressure again.
Having managed to follow this diet for 2-3 days, you should perceive an enormous change in your groin area. The hernia sac should be very soft and substantially smaller. Only now it is reasonable to treat hernia by use of a bandage (truss). The time is ripe to wear the truss. Maybe you will have to wait a little longer until you can use the truss. In my case it took 2 days until my hernia was „truss-qualified".
There is no more risk of an intestinal incarceration and that's after only 3 DAYS' DIETARY CHANGE!!!! This fact should encourage you to stand firm during the next months.

For Vegetarians

The vegetarians among you have to find appropriate alternatives for the respective meat meals keeping in mind that all processed, denaturised carbohydrates are forbidden Furthermore the most important instruction is still to be observed: Don't mix the food!
I doubt whether an exclusively vegetarian diet is reasonable, particularly as this kind of nutrition is contradictory to the laws of nature (see „chimpanzee").

Our responsibility towards animals should, however, not be diminished. In our society animals are tortured in a dishonourable and most disgusting manner. This must be improved by all means, without being able to change the human nature. You cannot consider a lion as a bad and cruel bastard because it eats living helpless, small and cute animals. It was not up to the lion's choice. It was just created that way by nature. If the lion ate salads every day, it would be highly appreciated by the vegetarians. The lion as vegetarian, however, would die very soon.

One my friends always fed his dog with bananas. Consequently the dog suffered from strong flatulence with terribly smelling breaking winds about every 30 seconds. The volume of the gases exceeded by far the dog's volume, which cannot be healthy.

Of course I do not know exactly which food is the best for promoting a healthy ageing of human beings. But I can tell you exactly which food is the best for healing hernia without surgery.

Putting on the Truss

You may only use the truss, if you continuously follow the before mentioned dietary plan. If you, however, return to your previous dietary habits, you must not wear the truss. In that case it could be more dangerous than useful.

The truss is put on in the morning upon getting up and is to be worn continuously until you go to bed in the evening. If you lie down (for example for a nap), the truss may be taken off. But as soon as you get up or sit up, you immediately have to put it on again. If you are lying on your back, the hernia sac should disappear. If not, you should consult a doctor. But I am sure that in most cases the hernia sac will return to the abdomen without being visible any longer, as long as the patients rest lying on their backs.

The material of the truss is of decisive importance! I have tried all available alternatives and innumerable trusses offered by the orthopaedics business.

In my view only a knitted scarf – no matter if it is finely or coarsely knitted – is suitable, as it is able to perfectly keep the groin in position for 24 hours a day. Furthermore it does not leave any pressure marks, being really comfortable. You have to wear it every day during the next 2 – 6 months. It will turn to be a part of you and must never be forgotten …. NOT EVEN ONCE!!!

As from this moment the hernia must NEVER AGAIN APPEAR. If you have to go to the toilet at night after having put off the truss, you have to press the groin area with your hands on your way to the toilet. The intestine must not be given the slightest chance of penetrating again the groin. I think this extremely radical measure has to be taken particularly during the first 6 weeks of treatment.

The truss must be worn under your clothes.... if necessary, a button of your trousers is left open or you have to wear a longer sweater to hide the truss. In summer you should wear wide cut Bermuda-shorts instead of small swimming trunks. I at least had to do so. Furthermore I use several trusses – if one of them needs to dry. Sometimes it's rather a bit bothersome to wear the truss all the times, but you can do everything while wearing it without any physical constraint. You can be in action, while your hernia is healing.

Having sex you should lie on your back, while your healthy partner is more active. As soon as you have put off the truss, you need to be careful as the groin must not be loaded without truss.

If you, however, insist of being the active partner during sex, you have to wear the truss during it. In that case you have to continuously care for the truss perfectly fitting all the time. I can hardly imagine that this is possible.

Should the groin rupture again now..... your therapy needs to be restarted. The groin will take time to stabilize and strengthen again. You should wait for at least 2 months before taking the risk. Otherwise the healing process would have to be started again. It would be bad for the tissue already formed………..

If you lie on your back, nothing can happen to your healing groin without truss.

.

In the following chapter the application of the truss is described in detail, taking a hernia on the left-hand side as example. Should you suffer from a hernia on the right-hand side, you of course have to execute the instructions in a mirror-inverted manner. Imagine (while looking at the photos) to be in front of a mirror. Then you only have to follow your mirror image and mirror each knot.

Instructions for Putting on the Truss:

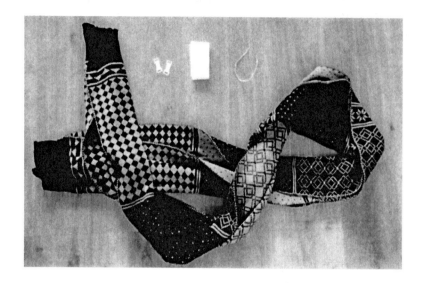

Material required for the truss:

1) An approx. 3m long **finely or coarsely knitted woollen scarf**!!!
In my view there no other material is more convenient for applying a perfect pressure bandage in the groin area.

2) A groin pad 5x9 cm and approx. 0,5 cm thick

3) Two clamps

4) A slightly flexible, coated wire.

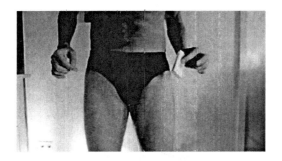

At first we use the groin pad.

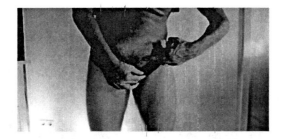

The groin pad is exactly positioned in longitudinal direction on the hernia.

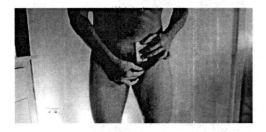

The groin pad is fixed in that position by the elastic tape of the shorts.

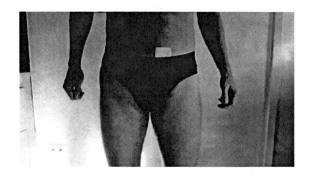

Now we have both hands free to apply the scarf.

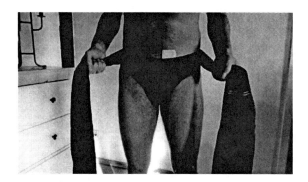

The scarf is put around the hip. The scarf's right end must be twice the length of the left end, as the right end is led between the legs to the back. In this example a hernia on the left-hand side is treated.

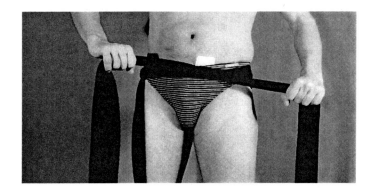

A normal knot is tied directly in front of the groin pad.

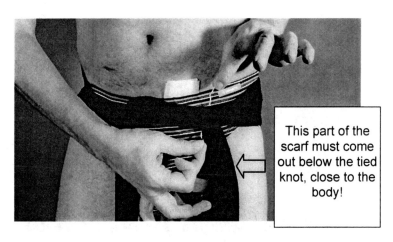

This part of the scarf must come out below the tied knot, close to the body!

Now the belt is knotted with a normal knot directly placed in front of the groin pad. To fix the knot, take the piece of wire and tie it around the scarf at the marked position.

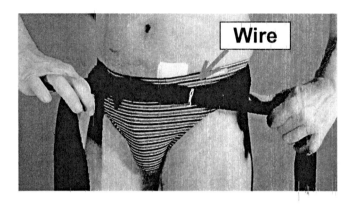

The wire stabilizes the part of the scarf that will be led between the legs.

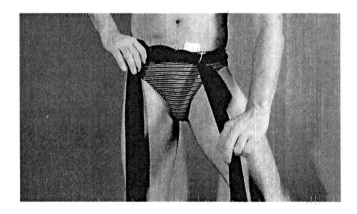

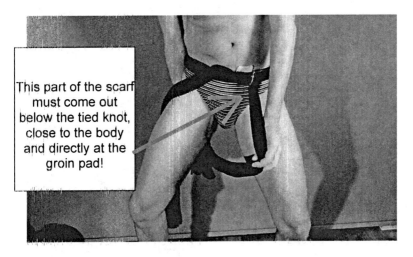

This part of the scarf must come out below the tied knot, close to the body and directly at the groin pad!

Now the scarf is led along the groin pad towards the back between the legs.

Take care that the end of the scarf, which will be led between the legs, is close to the body at the knot!!! That means: the scarf must be placed directly at the groin pad below the knot and not above the knot. Should the scarf's end come out above the knot, only insufficient pressure will be put on the groin pad. This is very important!!! – this part of the scarf being put between the legs puts the major pressure on the groin pad.

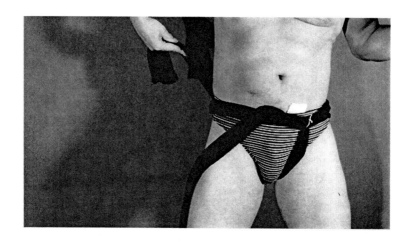

Both ends of the scarf are knotted aside the hip.

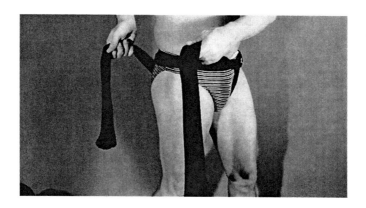

Tighten them (neither too loosely nor too strongly) in a normal knot aside the hip.

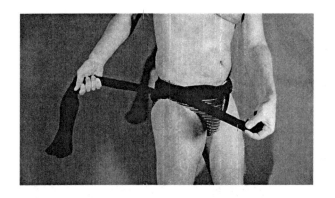

Pull the knot tightly aside the hip.

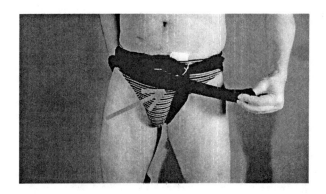

Both ends of the scarf are once again wrapped around the hip. Take again care of placing the scarf directly in front of the groin pad to put additional pressure on it (and consequently on the hernia opening).

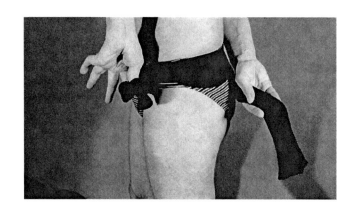

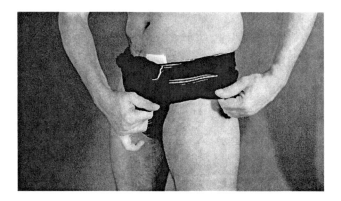

For the last time a normal knot is tightened aside the hip and pulled tight.

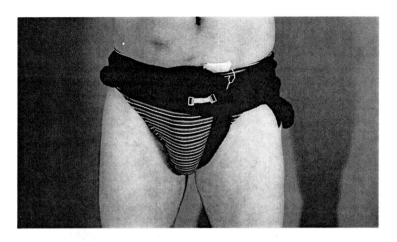

The two scarf ends are now fastened by the use of clamps. The more clamps are used, the more tight and safe the scarf arrangement will be.

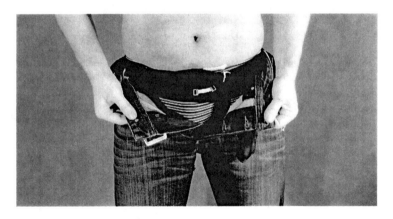

To be worn under the trousers; if necessary, one or two buttons must be left open.

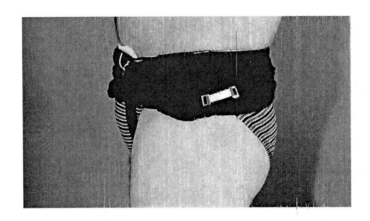

It should look like this on the left-hand side.

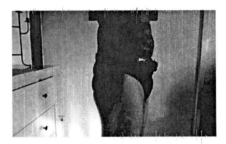

It should look like this on the other side.

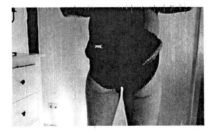

It should look like this from the back.

In no case use a truss bought in a shop!

A normal truss to be bought in an orthopaedic shop will never be helpful to you. It will even be more damaging than useful.

The truss technique - just being described - is suitable to perfectly stabilize the hernia opening (but only if the dietary instructions are followed). The truss can be designed individually. Independent from your stature, the described technique will always provide you with the perfect groin pressure bandage.

Wear the bandage (only in connection with the dietary change) for approx. 3-6 months. The groin will be returned to its normal position and the hernia can close. Due to its achieved strength you will not suffer from any discomfort in the groin area after 6 months. Furthermore a relapse is highly improbable (similar to a bone fracture, torn ligament or any other usual scar).

If you have stood firm for 2-4 months and your hernia has healed, I would nevertheless strongly recommend you to wear the truss for further months - just to be on the safe side (100% safety). You will see: after a very short time you will be able to put the truss on/off within a few seconds – even with blindfolded eyes.

Groin Pad

You can establish the groin pad on your own by using sheets of a kitchen roll (Zewa). Take 3-5 sheets and fold them 3 times. An approx. 6,5 x 12 cm sized groin pad will be formed.

If you use 5 sheets, take: 1 x 3 and 1 x 2 sheets …. Fold each of these packages three times and pile up these two flat pads. Thanks to this procedure a straight and thicker pad can be formed.

Use 3, 4 or 5 Zewa-sheets. The pad should be approx. 3-6 mm thick. I myself changed the thickness – depending on how tightly the belt has been tightened and depending on the activities you intend to do next.

Short Summary:

- Change the dietary and stand firm for approx. 2-6 months.

- Put on the truss every day so that the hernia sac will not appear again (and the hernia can close).

- Again: NEVER mix the food..... either only proteins (meat, eggs) or only raw food (fruits or salads).

- A minimum of 2-3 hours should go by between the meals. Following a meat meal it is even better not to eat during the next 4 hours.

- Always drink 20 min. before the meals. After the meals only drink in short sips.... or even better wait for 2-3 hours.

- Stand firm! You will be rid of your troubles in 2-4 months. During the 3 months' therapy your quality of life will not be reduced. On the contrary, you will live on a more healthy diet. But at the beginning you should refrain from extreme exertions.

- KEEP IN MIND: You save yourself an absolutely unnecessary operation with all its side effects as cut nerves, loss of the testicles, shrunken testicles, numbness, recovery pain, wound infections, trouble with the mesh, lifelong pain, risk of a general anaesthesia and all other complications which might occur during surgery.

- The meshes to be implanted are no alternative, but a proof of today's incompetent traditional medicine.

- The pressure put on the groin by the intestine can only be removed by adhering to the nutrition instructions!!!

- And the very last point: the risk of an intestinal incarceration should be decreased after 2-7 days.

- Only use the truss, if you adhere to the nutrition instructions!!!

Important Things to be Considered by All Means in Your Everyday Life

The **groin pad** can be established by using Zewa-sheets. 3 – 5 Zewa-sheets are to be folded three times so that an approx. 6,5 x 12 cm sized pad will come into being. Take 3-5 Zewa-sheets.

Do not take a shower, but have a bath - as you may lie during the bath. In case you do take a shower, you must not put off the truss!! You need a second truss, if the first is wet and need to dry. Alternatively you may take the shower while sitting in the shower basin.... You are not allowed to stand without truss.

If you need to go to the toilet at night, you have to take care of putting pressure with your hand on the hernia opening.

But it would be best to have an urine bottle next to your bed at night (at least during the first weeks) so that you needn't get up and stress your groin unnecessarily!!!

It's better to eat no sausage. Depending on its quality.... does it contain bread or any other ingredients which might lead to gas production in the intestine? No gas must be produced any longer!!! Buy all-natural products to be on the safe side.

Keep in mind...a usual meal (all components being mixed) leads to the production of approx. 15-20 litres of gas in the intestine.... no wonder that the groin will break somewhen ... and it will break................very certainly.... in case of each 3-4 person on earth.

Hernia on Both Sides

In case of hernia on both sides first put on the truss following the instructions given above. Concentrate only on one side.... it's the best to first treat the side with the larger hernia sac. You need a second groin pad to be put correspondingly on the second hernia. The first truss will already put some pressure on the second hernia, which, is, however, insufficient. It is necessary to put another scarf around the hip, which it is to be placed in such a way that also the second hernia is correctly covered and stabilized.

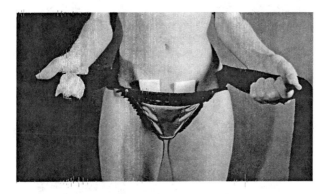

In a first step you have to place the two groin pads on both hernia openings, afterwards put the scarf around the hip.

Now you will exactly follow the instructions given above:

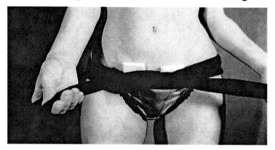

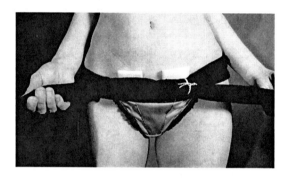

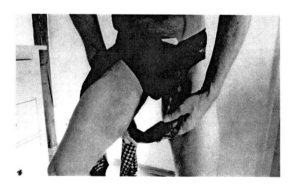

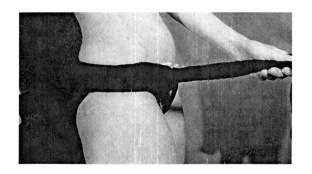

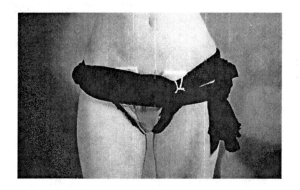

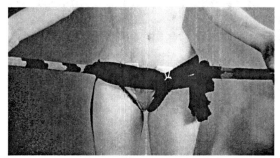

Now a second scarf is put around the hip.

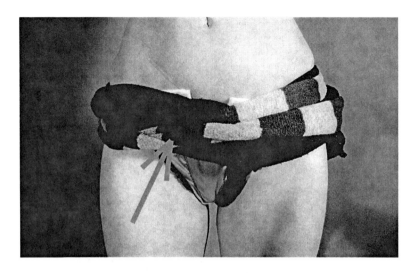

In addition to the first scarf the second scarf is once put around the hip and knotted (normal knot) directly in front of the second groin pad (see arrow). This second truss is fixed by the first truss and cannot slip. Take care that it is positioned at the second groin pad (see arrow) below the first truss (directly on the hernia, see arrow). Thus pressure is simultaneously put on the second groin pad by both trusses (see arrow).

It does not look highly professional. But if you really suffer from hernia on both sides, there is no better solution. Applying this technique, both hernia will be perfectly treated.

The truss may only be used if you adhere to the dietary plan!

Further Examples of Meals:

I'll come to the point right away: the more uniform the daily dietary plan is, the more successful will be the healing process of your groin. Therefore don't be surprised that the meals will be repeated several times. That's not due to a lack of fantasy, but pure intention. In my view it would be the best to eat only one single type of food (for example: only oranges and orange juice) during the whole time of treatment (approx. 2-4 months). But this is neither somewhat realistic nor fun.

During the dietary change you sometimes might suffer from slight stomach ache. Probably your body first has to get used to the new, healthy dietary or the stomach ache is a sign of detoxication.

Monday:

Breakfast:

2   cups of filter coffee with little condensed milk (**by no means** sugar is to be added)
3 – 4   Medjool dates
1   banana

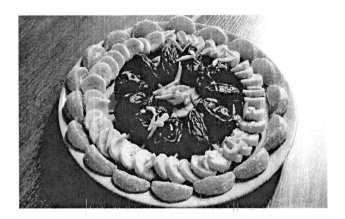

A delicious breakfast for 3 persons is shown on this photo. It is very nourishing, filling and taste nice with coffee. This breakfast makes you forget the rolls bought from the baker's.

Lunch:

If you are travelling a lot on business, you should have a quick meal in form of a banana, Medjool dates or figs.

Should you have enough time, prepare a Greek farmer salad:

1 – 2	tomatoes (cut into small pieces)
¼	cucumber (cut into small pieces as well)
4	olives
1	avocado (small)
½	paprika
60 g	feta cheese (alternatively 80 g mozzarella)
2 – 3	soup spoons of olive oil
1	pinch of herbs of Provence
1	pinch of salt (preferably: Himalaya-salt)

Supper:

Have a drink before supper, preferably water or freshly squeezed orange juice/carrot juice. Afterwards you should wait for approx. 15-25 min. before starting to eat.

200 g – 450 g	fried boneless chicken breast (without side dishes)
approx. 50 g	herb butter or butter

Use by no means sauces or other side dishes. Slightly season the meat. The less spices, the better. During supper you may only drink max. 0.2l, for example of wine. But it would be best not to drink at all during the meals. After a meal 2-3 hours should always go by before drinking.

Tuesday:

Breakfast:

1 – 2	cups of filter coffee (or tea) without sugar, maybe little condensed milk
2	medium-sized grated carrots
1	squeezed banana
15	raisins
1	pinch of almond slivers
1 – 2	soup spoons of condensed milk or cream

Mix all ingredients.

Lunch:

125 g	strawberries
100 g	blueberries or raspberries
1	banana
100 g	grapes
1 – 2	Medjool dates
1 – 2	soup spoons of condensed milk or cream

As far as necessary, cut all ingredients and mix them.

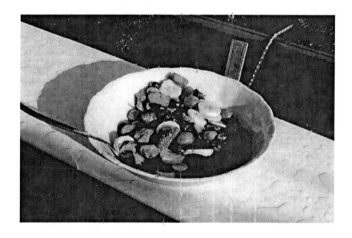

Always keep in mind: also in case of very delicious and healthy food, it is important to remember: the less, the better.

Supper:

First have some drink, preferably up to 0,5 l water or freshly squeezed carrot juice respectively orange juice. Afterwards you should wait for approx. 15-25 min. before starting to eat.

250 g – 450 g	mince (pork or beef or mixed) as meat balls; by no means add soaked bread or flour. Only the meat with an egg, some olive oil and slightly seasoned. No onions!
1	egg
50 g	herb butter

Wednesday:

Breakfast:

1 – 2 cups of filter coffee (or tea) without sugar
1 - 2 bananas
2 – 4 Medjool dates
1 – 2 dried figs

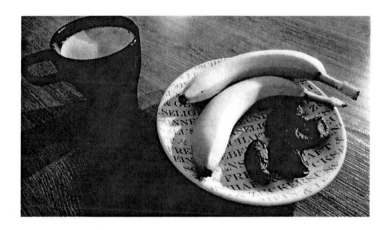

This breakfast for 3 persons is quickly prepared, very nourishing, filling and tastes nice. Stand firm and do not go shopping at the baker's.

Lunch: (1.00pm to 7.00pm depending on your personal rhythm)

First have some drink. Afterwards wait for approx. 15-25 min. before starting to eat.

Omelette:

2 – 4	eggs
50 g	feta cheese
2 – 4	soup spoons of olive oil

Season it!

Supper:

First have some drink, preferably freshly squeezed carrot juice or orange juice. Drink slowly, insalivating the juice. If you drank too quickly and too much in one go, the healing process of your groin would be endangered.

250 – 450 g	rib eye steak
40 – 80 g	herb butter
3 – 5	soup spoons of olive oil

Season cautiously.

You may have 0,2 litres of red wine.

The Advantage of Hernia: It Is Visible!

Contrary to all other diseases hernia has the big advantage of being visible. Miracle healers, blithering idiots and charlatans cannot state to have healed hernia, as they can do in case of many other illnesses. No naturopath, miracle healer or homeopath dares to treat hernia. Only the traditional doctor with his scalpel does. But who wants to be operated? But why do the charlatans dare to treat almost all other diseases? No doubt.... Nobody can find out at once if the patient has been healed or not. In case of hernia, however, it is visible immediately whether the buckle in the groin area has disappeared or not. A miracle healer will treat you, no matter from which kind of illness you are suffering. Or he will cheat on you by performing a game in cooperation with another person who first pretends to be ill, followed by his subsequent healing. The miracle healer will, however, refuse to treat your hernia as in that case he has to put his cards on the table....

But you may benefit from this fact, as any improvement or deterioration of your hernia is revealed by the size of the hernia sac every day. If you adhere to the instructions given in this book, your hernia should improve with the hernia sac becoming smaller every day. This continuous progress in turn will motivate you to stand firm until your groin has been entirely healed.
It would be great if you observed the instructions so that your hernia could heal. But you have to do a lot to achieve this aim. The dietary plan will be a real challenge

for many readers. But there is no getting around it! Surgery is the only alternative! The truss will be a part of you for about 4 months, but you will get used to it within short and put it on/off within seconds.

The truss needs to be worn at all times (except during lying) – while you are working, getting exercise (also while you are swimming; you possibly need a second truss), while you are passing the security zone at the airport (during the body check the truss under your clothes may cause a stir), and so on.

Stand firm for a few months and you will get rid of your hernia … no matter how long you had been suffering from it.

Adhere to these detailed instructions. If you additionally use the further contents of the book as motivational thoughts, I would highly appreciate it.

If you follow the nutrition rules of this book, you may benefit from its positive side effect: you will not break winds any longer. Should gases still be produced, your daily food is most probably wrong. By all means, do not deviate from this dietary plan! A small piece of bread could seriously endanger the healing process. In my view a fart is already the first step towards a disease.

It's a kind of acoustic alarm of your body, comparable with the alarm given by a car in case of missing oil. Should you ignore the alarm and continue going by car without refilling oil, the motor will soon be damaged.

Gases will no more be produced in the intestine, as long as you follow this dietary plan. Gas production in the intestine is equal to an internal pressure put on the groin. Thus the groin is exposed to a permanent load. Constant dripping wears the rock away – accordingly the gas-filled intestine will find its way to the outside. That's exactly how hernia comes into being (at least in most cases):

During the digestion of a single meal in which food was mixed (that means carbohydrates and proteins) up to 18 litres of gas are produced in the intestine. If this entire quantity of gas was discharged in form of flatulence, we would certainly break winds all day. But most of the intestine's gas is absorbed by the blood and led into the air via the lungs and the breathing air. As you can easily imagine, this way of gas removal takes far longer than breaking winds.

In case of very strong digestion processes (and this will be applicable for most people) the gas is produced faster than being discharged by breathing air. This process is called flatulence.

18 litres of gas are quite a lot. The intestine is extremely bloated and the physical forces impacting the groin are enormous.

With this book you will always be one or several step(s) ahead of all hernia specialists.

It's up to you now.

Take your chance!

„Das Weltall und die Dummheit der Menschen sind unendlich... wobei ich mir beim Weltall nicht ganz sicher bin."

Albert Einstein

The universe and the stupidity of human beeing are infinitely... but i am not so sure with the universe

Albert Einstein

CPSIA information can be obtained
at www.ICGtesting.com
Printed in the USA
FSOW02n0813100118
43254FS